Cecelia's Marketplace

Easy 30 Day Gluten-Free Diet

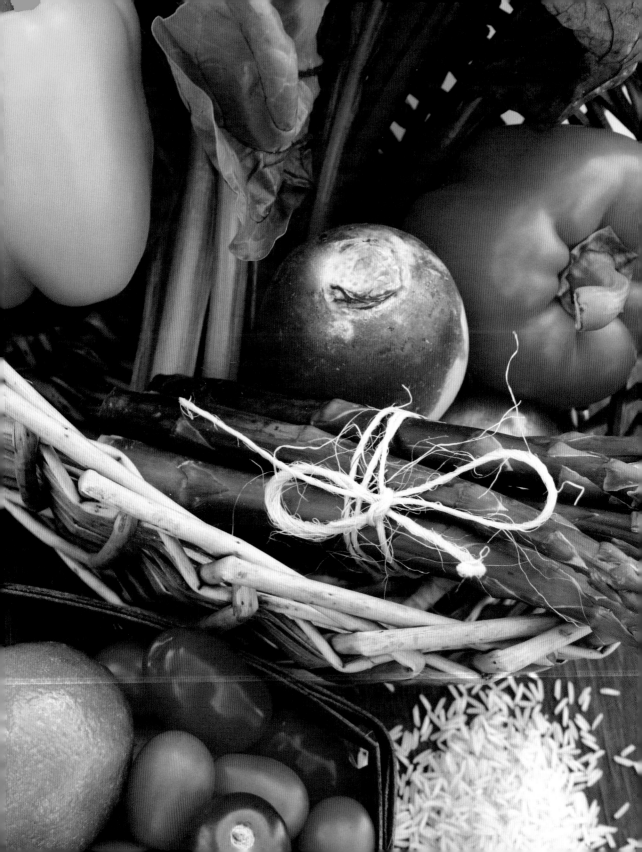

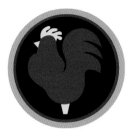

Cecelia's Marketplace

Easy 30 Day Gluten-Free Diet

DR. MARA MATISON

khP

Kal-Haven Publishing

Cecelia's Marketplace Easy 30 Day Gluten-Free Diet
Dr. Mara Matison

khP
Kal-Haven Publishing
P.O. Box 20383
Kalamazoo, MI 49019 U.S.A.

ISBN 978-0-9831659-1-0

Printed in the United States of America

CONTENTS

DISCLAIMER

This book is for informational purposes only and should be used as an aide to guide the consumer in the right direction when starting a gluten-free diet. The content of this book is not medical advice. The author, Cecelia's Marketplace, and Kal-Haven Publishing shall have neither liability, nor responsibility to any person or entity with respect to gluten ingestion or any health consequence from the gluten-free diet described in this book.

Every effort has been made to make this book as complete and accurate as possible. However, there may be errors, both typographical and in content.

Food companies and manufacturers indicate that product ingredients may change periodically; therefore, the consumer always needs to check the ingredients on the manufacturers' labels before consuming their products. For further information on a gluten-free diet, please consult your physician.

Any product brand mentioned in this book does not imply endorsement of that product by the author, Cecelia's Marketplace, nor Kal-Haven Publishing.

Recipes using raw or undercooked eggs, meat, poultry, fish or seafood should be avoided by infants, the elderly, pregnant women, convalescents and anyone suffering from a chronic illness.

INTRODUCTION

Are you wondering if gluten may be affecting your health? Thinking about trying a gluten-free diet? Not sure how to start a gluten-free diet? *Cecelia's Marketplace Easy 30 Day Gluten-Free Diet* plan is the perfect resource to help you get started.

Gluten, the protein found in wheat, rye and barley, is quickly gaining attention in the media. Researchers are finding that gluten may be responsible for a variety of symptoms, ranging from abdominal pain, anemia, osteoporosis and unexplained weight loss to panic attacks, migraines and depression.

Maybe you have a family member that was just diagnosed with gluten intolerance or celiac disease. Maybe you are the type of person that likes to try something new and healthy. Maybe you want to see why so many Hollywood stars and professional athletes swear by a gluten-free diet. Whatever the reason may be, this book will help you get started.

Unlike most diets, *Cecelia's Marketplace Easy 30 Day Gluten-Free Diet* is not designed for weight loss, but to determine if gluten is negatively affecting your body. This book makes starting a gluten-free diet easy and headache free. It includes step-by-step instructions, a 30 day gluten-free menu plan, a mini gluten-free grocery shopping guide, gluten-free kitchen & cooking tips, and 30 delicious gluten-free dinner recipes!

NOTE TO THE READER

Cecelia's Marketplace Easy 30 Day Gluten-Free Diet is designed to guide you through a gluten-free diet for the next 30 days. To better understand how to use the information in this book, please read the following notes.

This diet is not intended for weight loss. All of our recipes are meant to serve two (150 lb.) persons. You may consume as little or as much of the recommended meals as you wish. For larger appetites, you may double the recipes. All recipes use US standard measurements. All spoon measurements are level. Tablespoons (Tbsp.) are considered to be 15 ml.. Teaspoons (tsp.) are considered to be 5 ml..

To make your gluten-free journey easier, share with your co-workers, friends and family members what your goal is for the next 30 days. Who knows, maybe one of them will be interested in trying the diet with you. For additional support, you may consider joining a local gluten-free support group where you can learn gluten-free tips, recipes and information on gluten-free restaurants in your area. For a list of gluten-free support group organizations, please see page 19.

During your 30-day gluten-free diet, the most important guideline is to consume foods that are strictly gluten-free. Sometimes even consuming a bite of a pizza or half of a sandwich can cause a noticeable setback in your health. Some individuals that have celiac disease or gluten intolerance are so sensitive to gluten, that even a bread crumb can cause an adverse reaction.

To help you grocery shop, we have compiled a *Mini Gluten-Free Grocery Shopping Guide* (pages 167-185) that lists specific brand names of products that are gluten-free. These foods are popular products found in most nationwide grocery stores. We recommend that you shop for these specific brands, otherwise you may run the risk of consuming products that contain gluten. For our full list of thousands of gluten-free grocery products, you may be interested in purchasing *Cecelia's Marketplace Gluten-Free Grocery Shopping Guide.* Order online: www.CeceliasMarketplace.com

We have also supplied an easy reference chart on page 21 that lists *Safe vs. Unsafe Foods* to consume on a gluten-free diet. A good rule of thumb to remember is that: all fresh fruits & vegetables, fresh eggs, fresh meat, poultry and seafood (non-marinated and unseasoned) are gluten-free.

Cecelia's Marketplace Easy 30 Day Gluten-Free Diet includes a daily menu plan that outlines what foods to eat for breakfast, lunch, dinner and also for snacks. **It is highly advised that those foods that are marked with a ✓ symbol be selected from our *Mini Gluten-Free Grocery Shopping Guide* on page 167.**

If you would prefer to skip a recommended meal option, you may make a substitution using the other choices we have listed. Breakfast choices are listed on page 26, lunch choices on page 27, dinner choices on page 28 and snack choices on page 30. Keep in mind that we have designed this plan so that your options are continuously rotating, you get a wide variety of nutrients and flavors, and to eliminate monotonous meals.

The next 30 days will be an exciting journey where you will learn how to prepare, eat and live a gluten-free lifestyle.

Good luck, be patient and enjoy the journey!

ACKNOWLEDGEMENTS

Thank you to my husband Dainis, for his encouragement, support, artistic photography, page layout, and design ideas; to my meticulous editing team of Caroline, Lauma, Ligita, Lija, Lily, Mik, Ray and Tina; Savannah Studios for the amazing photoshooting facility; my fabulous tasting panel; and Kal-Haven Publishing.

ABOUT THE AUTHOR

Dr. Mara Matison is the founder of Cecelia's Marketplace, one of the top gluten-free resource companies on the market today. She has authored over 11 books and is known for her nationwide best selling *Gluten-Free Grocery Shopping Guide* and *Gluten-Free International Classics Cookbook* series. Living with celiac disease herself, Mara has become an expert on living a gluten-free lifestyle and preparing tasty & flavorful gluten-free meals.

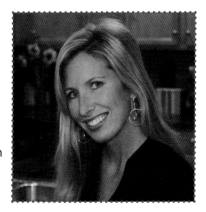

Besides being hard at work compiling helpful gluten-free resources, she spends her days as a private practice dentist. She earned her Doctor of Dental Surgery degree from University of Detroit Mercy and Bachelor of Arts degree in Psychology from Villanova University. She has been practicing dentistry for over 10 years and thoroughly enjoys both the medical field as well as publishing books on how to make gluten-free living easier.

Mara is a member of the American Dental Association, Michigan Dental Association, Celiac Disease Foundation, Celiac Sprue Association and Gluten Intolerance Group.

Being very active in sports her entire life, Mara continues to play competitive volleyball and tennis. Her hobbies include painting, swimming, and organic gardening.

WHAT IS GLUTEN?

Gluten is a protein that is most commonly found in wheat, rye, and barley. It is found in most cereals, breads, pastas, soups, and pizza crusts. It may also be hidden in foods such as seasonings, salad dressings, sauces, additives, fillers and natural flavors. People that have celiac disease, gluten intolerance, or gluten sensitivity may suffer from a wide array of adverse symptoms after ingesting gluten.

WHAT IS GLUTEN INTOLERANCE?

Gluten intolerance, or sometimes referred to as gluten sensitivity, is when an individual develops adverse health symptoms when ingesting gluten. Though some of these symptoms may be similar to celiac disease, this condition has not advanced to the severity of intestinal lining damage. Gluten intolerance can be effectively managed with a gluten-free diet. Some experts believe that gluten intolerance may be as common as 1 in every 20 Americans.

WHAT IS CELIAC DISEASE?

Celiac disease is an inherited autoimmune disorder. When people with celiac disease consume foods containing gluten, an immune reaction occurs and the villi (the small hair-like projections) of the small intestine become damaged. Without healthy villi the body is unable to absorb nutrients and becomes malnourished. There is no cure for celiac disease, however it can be managed effectively with a gluten-free diet. Studies show that approximately 1 in 133 Americans have celiac disease[1].

[1] University of Maryland Medical Center, Dr. Alessio Fasano, 2003 Archives of Internal Medicine

POSSIBLE SYMPTOMS

Maintaining a strict gluten-free diet may help alleviate most symptoms of gluten intolerance and celiac disease. After gluten is completely eliminated from the diet, symptoms usually start to disappear within a few weeks.

Symptoms of gluten intolerance and celiac disease vary from person to person. Below is a list of possible symptoms that may be related to gluten ingestion.

Abdominal Pain
Acid Reflux
Anemia
Bloating
Bone Loss
Bone Pain
Constipation
Delayed Growth In Children
Dental Enamel Defects
Depression
Diarrhea
Fatigue/Loss Of Energy
Hair Loss
Heart Palpitations

Infertility
Irritability
Joint Pain
Malnutrition
Migraine Headaches
Muscle Cramps
Painful Itchy Bumps On The Skin
Panic Attacks
Recurrent Miscarriage
Restless Legs
Seizures
Tingling Of Hands Or Feet
Unexplained Weight Loss Or Gain
Vitamin & Mineral Deficiencies

TESTING OPTIONS

Here are a few testing options for celiac disease and gluten intolerance.

AT HOME:
  At-Home Gluten Sensitivity Gene Test:
  EnteroLab   *www.enterolab.com*

  At-Home Food Intolerance Stool Sample Test:
  EnteroLab   *www.enterolab.com*

AT THE DOCTOR'S OFFICE:
  Celiac Genetic Blood Test:
  Celiac Genetic Assessment HLA DQ2/DQ8

  Celiac Disease Serology Blood Test:
  Anti-human tissue transglutaminase (Hu-tTG) IgA recombinant antigen,
  Anti-endomysial IgA, Total serum IgA, Anti-gliadin IgA, Anti-gliadin IgG

  Endoscopy Procedure:
  A biopsy of the small intestinal lining is performed by a gastroenterologist to
  confirm damaged intestinal villi, signifying celiac disease.

RESEARCH CENTERS:
  Columbia University - Celiac Disease Center
  University of Chicago - Celiac Disease Center
  University of Maryland - Center for Celiac Research

SUPPORT

Ask for support: Speak to your family and friends and describe to them the diet you will be doing for the next 30 days. Explain to them the foods that you can and cannot eat. Ask that they support you on your endeavour.

Journey with a friend: Ask a friend or family member to join you in trying this gluten-free diet. It is always easier when you have someone with whom you can share your journey.

Find local support: You may be surprised how many local celiac disease and gluten intolerance support groups are available. Most local support groups have monthly meetings or get togethers. Here you can find answers to questions, learn the do's and don'ts of a gluten-free diet, learn about local gluten-free restaurants, share gluten-free recipes, sample gluten-free products and meet others that are living a gluten-free lifestyle.

Nationwide Celiac Disease/Gluten Intolerance Support Groups:

CDF - Celiac Disease Foundation *www.celiac.org*
CSA - Celiac Sprue Association *www.csaceliacs.info*
GIG - Gluten Intolerance Group *www.gluten.net*
NFCA - National Foundation for Celiac Awareness *www.celiaccentral.org*

GLUTEN-FREE KITCHEN TIPS

It is very important prior to preparing a gluten-free meal to clean the cooking area, including: kitchen surfaces, pots, pans, utensils and any other items being used. Bread crumbs, flour particles and other gluten containing foods left in the cooking area can potentially contaminate a gluten-free meal. Here are some tips to help prevent gluten contamination:

- Use an uncontaminated or new sponge to wash all working surfaces with soap and water.
- Clean and inspect pots, pans, utensils, cutting boards and other kitchenware for gluten residue.
- Use clean kitchen hand towels.
- If grilling, place aluminum foil over the grilling surface.
- Avoid using wooden utensils. Gluten residue can stay embedded in wooden utensils and cutting boards.
- Use a separate toaster for gluten-free bread, rice cakes, etc.. If a separate toaster is not available, toast your bread on a warm frying pan.
- Do not deep fry foods in contaminated oil (e.g. from breaded chicken wings, breaded chicken tenders, mozzarella sticks).
- Use squeeze bottle mayonnaise, mustard, ketchup, peanut butter, jelly/jam, butter/margarine and other condiments to prevent cross-contamination.

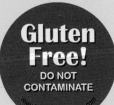

SAFE VS. UNSAFE FOODS

GLUTEN-FREE	POSSIBLE HIDDEN GLUTEN	CONTAINS GLUTEN
Amaranth	Bouillon Cubes	Barley
Arrowroot	Broth	Barley Malt
Beans	Caramel Color	Batter
Buckwheat	Caramel Flavoring	Beer
Carob	Dextrins	Bran
Coconut	Emulsifiers	Breading
Corn	Flavoring	Bulgur
Cornstarch	Food Starch	Couscous
Distilled Alcohol	Gravy	Hydrolyzed Wheat Protein
Distilled Vinegar	Hydrolyzed Protein	Hydrolyzed Wheat Starch
Eggs	Hydrolyzed Vegetable Protein	Kamut
Flax	Maltodextrin	Malt
Fresh Fruits & Vegetables	Miso	Malt Vinegar
Fresh Meat	Modified Food Starch	Oats*
Fresh Poultry	Natural Flavoring	Orzo
Fresh Seafood	Salad Dressings	Rye
Lentils	Sauces	Semolina
Milk	Soups	Spelt
Millet	Soy Sauce	Triticale
Nuts	Spice Blends	Triticum Vulgaris
Oil (Canola, Olive, Vegetable)	Stabilizers	Wheat
Potatoes	Teriyaki Sauce	Wheat Flour
Pure Herbs & Spices		Wheat Germ Oil
Quinoa		Wheat Gluten
Rice		
Sorghum		* Certified Gluten-Free oats are safe
Soy		
Tapioca		
Teff		

DINING OUT

Although dining out is not recommended during this diet, we realize that it may be inevitable. To be best prepared, here are some gluten-free dining out strategies:

- Choose a restaurant with a gluten-free menu. For a list of these restaurants please see below.
- If you are dining out at a restaurant that does not have a gluten-free menu, explain your dietary needs to your wait staff. Ask to speak with the chef to see if there are any naturally gluten-free foods that can be prepared for you.
- Go to restaurants at times when they are not very busy, to prevent cross contamination of your meal.

Cecelia's Marketplace offers a **Gluten-Free Dining Out Card** that helps explain to the wait staff & chef what foods you can and cannot have.

Order online: **www.CeceliasMarketplace.com**

CAUTION - Food Allergy

I have a severe food allergy/intolerance to GLUTEN. gluten is the protein found in wheat, rye and barley. I will become very sick if I ingest even the smallest amount of gluten

PLEASE wash & clean all cooking surfaces, grills, pots, pans, cutting boards and cooking utensils to remove any gluten residue before cooking my meal.

DO NOT include/use any flour based, in the sauce or marinade, and/or other gluten containing items such as chicken wings, chicken tenders, breaded fish, mozzarella sticks, etc.

The BACK OF THIS CARD has a list of foods I CAN & CANNOT have.

*please show this card to the chef that will be preparing my meal

Nationwide Restaurant Chains Offering Gluten-Free Menus:

Austin Grill	Legal Sea Foods Restaurant
Bertucci's Italian Restaurant	Mama Fu's Asian House
Biaggi's Ristorante Italiano	Mitchell's Fish Market
Bonefish Grill	Ninety Nine 99
Bugaboo Creek Steak House	Old Spaghetti Factory
Carino's Italian	Outback Steakhouse
Carrabba's Italian Grill	P.F. Chang's China Bistro
Charlie Brown's Steakhouse	Pei Wei Asian Diner
Cheeseburger In Paradise Bar & Grill	Pizza Fusion
Claim Jumper Restaurants	The Melting Pot
Daily Grill	Village Tavern
Fleming's Prime Steakhouse	Weber Grill Restaurant
Garlic Jim's Famous Gourmet Pizza	Wildfire Steaks, Chops & Seafood
Lee Roy Selmon's	Z' Tejas Southwestern Grill

This book is dedicated to all those in search of an easy step-by-step gluten-free diet plan.

GLUTEN-FREE
MEAL OPTIONS

BREAKFAST CHOICES

All fresh fruits and eggs are gluten-free. Certain brands of bacon, ham, hashbrowns, margarine, salsa, sausage, and yogurt may contain gluten. Most regular cereals contain gluten. Please use the **Mini Gluten-Free Grocery Shopping Guide on pg. 167** for specific gluten-free brands that you can enjoy.

Banana Blueberry Smoothie
Banana Pineapple Smoothie
Cream of Rice Cereal
Eggs, Bacon & Hashbrowns
Eggs, Ham & Hashbrowns
Eggs, Sausage & Hashbrowns
Fresh Fruit & Gluten-Free Toast
Fresh Fruit & Yogurt
Gluten-Free Cereal & Milk w/Banana Slices
Scrambled Eggs w/Salsa & Hashbrowns

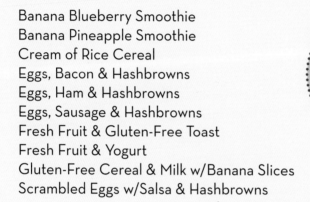

Smoothie Recipes pg. 158

Olive oil is a healthy option for frying eggs, hashbrowns or other foods.

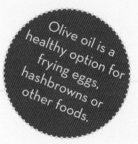

Intolerant to regular milk? Try almond, coconut, rice or soy milk.

LUNCH CHOICES

All fresh salad greens are gluten-free. Certain brands of chips, deli meats, salad dressings, and soups may contain gluten. Regular bread, crackers and croutons contain gluten. Please use the **Mini Gluten-Free Grocery Shopping Guide on pg. 167** for specific gluten-free brands that you can enjoy.

Caesar Salad
Chicken w/Rice Soup
Garden Salad w/Italian Dressing
Garden Salad w/Ranch Dressing
Garden Salad w/Raspberry Vinaigrette Dressing
Greek Salad
Ham Sandwich
New England Clam Chowder
Roast Beef Sandwich
Salami Sandwich
Split Pea w/Ham Soup
Tomato Soup
Tuna Fish Sandwich
Turkey Sandwich
Vegetable Soup

All lunches include chips. Gluten-free chips are listed on pg. 171

Greek Salad: lettuce, feta cheese, olives, red onion slices & greek dressing.

Caesar Salad: romaine lettuce, parmesan cheese & caesar dressing.

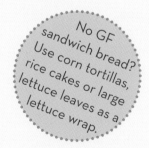
No GF sandwich bread? Use corn tortillas, rice cakes or large lettuce leaves as a lettuce wrap.

Need GF Croutons? Cut GF bread into small cubes, toss in olive oil & bake at 300 degrees for 10 min.

DINNER CHOICES

Each dinner meal includes a recipe. The recipe page numbers are listed below. All fresh fruits & vegetables, fresh eggs, fresh meat, poultry and seafood that is non-marinated and unseasoned are gluten free. Certain brands of BBQ sauce, teriyaki sauce, french fries and marinara sauce may contain gluten. Regular hamburger buns and pasta contain gluten. Please use the **Mini Gluten-Free Grocery Shopping Guide on pg. 167** for specific gluten-free brands that you can enjoy.

Baked Chicken w/Chimichurri Sauce, Mashed Potatoes & Green Beans, *pg. 96*
BBQ Chicken w/Oven Baked Fries & Corn on the Cob, *pg. 88*
BBQ Pork Chops w/Baked Beans & Corn on the Cob, *pg. 72*
BBQ Pork Chops w/Mashed Potatoes & Corn on the Cob, *pg. 120*
Beef Tacos w/Fresh Salsa & Avocado Cubes, *pg. 44*
Cheeseburger w/Oven Baked Fries, *pg. 104*
Chicken Pasta Primavera in Garlic Sauce, *pg. 136*
Chicken Tenders & Steamed Artichoke w/White Rice, *pg. 148*
Chicken Tenders w/Oven Baked Fries & Steamed Artichoke, *pg. 56*
Fish & Chips w/Coleslaw, *pg. 144*
Fish Tacos w/Fresh Salsa & Avocado Cubes, *pg. 100*
Gluten-Free Pasta w/Beef Marinara Sauce & Zucchini, *pg. 52*
Gluten-Free Spaghetti w/Beef Marinara Sauce & Zucchini, *pg. 92*
Grilled Lamb Chops, Vegetables & Brown Rice w/Chimichurri Sauce, *pg. 112*
Grilled Salmon w/Lemon Dill Sauce, Steamed Snow Peas & Brown Rice, *pg. 36*
Grilled Shish Kebobs & Quinoa w/Garlic Sauce, *pg. 76*
Grilled Steak, Vegetables & Brown Rice w/Chimichurri Sauce, *pg. 64*
Grilled Steak & Vegetables w/Sweet Potato Fries, *pg. 128*
Grilled Steak w/Baked Potato & Broccoli, *pg. 152*
Pan-Seared Salmon w/Fresh Salsa & Mango Served Over Brown Rice, *pg. 132*
Pan-Seared Salmon w/GF Teriyaki Sauce, Steamed Broccoli & White Rice, *pg. 68*
Pan-Seared Tilapia in Garlic Sauce w/Asparagus & White Rice, *pg. 84*
Pan-Seared Tilapia w/Fresh Salsa, Mango Slices & Brown Rice, *pg. 60*
Potato Encrusted Tilapia, Green Beans & White Rice w/Lemon Dill Sauce, *pg. 108*

DINNER CHOICES

Sautéed Shrimp, Onions & Red Peppers w/Garlic Sauce Over Quinoa, *pg. 48*
Shrimp Kebobs w/Grilled Vegetables & Quinoa, *pg. 124*
Stir-Fried Chicken & Vegetables in GF Teriyaki Sauce w/Brown Rice, *pg. 40*
Teriyaki Chicken w/Sautéed Green Beans & Brown Rice, *pg. 116*
Turkey Burger w/Sautéed Onions & Mushrooms and Sweet Potato Fries, *pg. 80*
Turkey Tacos w/Fresh Salsa & Avocado Cubes, *pg. 140*

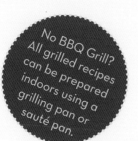

No BBQ Grill? All grilled recipes can be prepared indoors using a grilling pan or sauté pan.

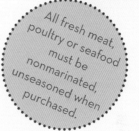

Sauce Recipes: pg. 159-161

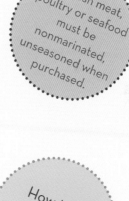

All fresh meat, poultry or seafood must be nonmarinated, unseasoned when purchased.

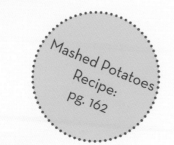

Mashed Potatoes Recipe: pg. 162

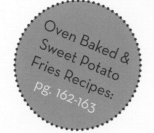

Oven Baked & Sweet Potato Fries Recipes: pg. 162-163

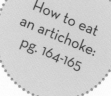

How to eat an artichoke: pg. 164-165

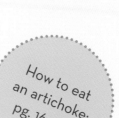

SNACK CHOICES

All fresh fruits & vegetables and natural applesauce are gluten-free. Many snacks contain gluten. Please be sure to use the **Mini Gluten-Free Grocery Shopping Guide on pg. 167** when shopping for ALL the snacks listed below.

HEALTHY:
Apple Slices w/Caramel Dip
Applesauce
Carrot Sticks w/Ranch Dip
Fresh Fruit
Fruit Cocktail Cup
Mandarin Orange Cup
Snack Bar
Sorbet
Yogurt

For optimal health, try to minimize your sweet and salty snack intake.

SALTY:
Corn Chips
Popcorn
Rice Chips
Roasted & Salted Nuts
Potato Chips
Veggie Chips

For specific brand name gluten-free snacks please see pg. 167

SWEET:
Candy Bar
Ice Cream
Jello
Popsicle
Pudding

DRINK CHOICES

All 100% fruit & vegetable juices are naturally gluten-free. All distilled alcohol is gluten-free. All wine and champagne/sparkling wine made in the US is gluten-free. Certain brands of carbonated beverages may contain gluten. Please use the **Mini Gluten-Free Grocery Shopping Guide on pg. 167** for specific gluten-free brands that you can enjoy.

JUICE:
Apple
Cranberry
CranApple
CranPomegranate
CranGrape
Grape
Lemonade
Orange
Pineapple
Tomato

COFFEE & TEA:
Caffeinated Coffee
Caffeinated Tea
Decaf Coffee
Decaf Tea

CARBONATED BEVERAGES:
Club Soda
Diet Soda Pop
Seltzer
Soda Pop
Tonic Water

ALCOHOLIC BEVERAGES:
Champagne
Cider
Distilled Liquor
Gluten-Free Beer
Wine

Try to minimize or eliminate alcohol intake during your 30 day diet.

Remember to stay hydrated... drink at least 8 glasses of water a day!

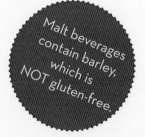

Malt beverages contain barley, which is NOT gluten-free.

30 DAY
GLUTEN-FREE
DIET PLAN

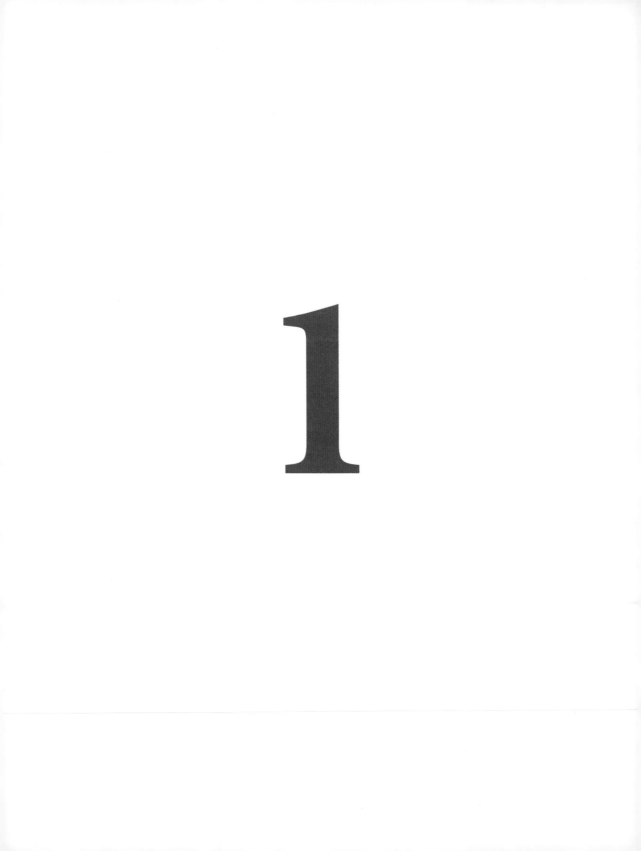

1

TODAY'S MENU: **Day 1**

BREAKFAST
....
Eggs, Bacon ✓ & Hashbrowns ✓

SNACK
(optional)
....
Orange Slices

LUNCH
....
Garden Salad with Italian Dressing ✓
& Corn Chips ✓

SNACK
(optional)
....
Popcorn ✓

DINNER
....
Grilled Salmon with Lemon Dill Sauce,
Steamed Snow Peas & Brown Rice

Fresh
pineapple
contains bromelain,
a natural enzyme,
which aids in
digestion.

SNACK
(optional)
....
Fresh Pineapple Slices

✓ Please make sure this product is gluten-free.
For specific brand name gluten-free products please see page 167.

GRILLED SALMON
with lemon dill sauce, steamed snow peas & brown rice

SERVES 2

brown rice (see package for serving size)
2 medium salmon fillets, with skin
2 cups snow peas

Lemon Dill Sauce:
2 Tbsp. freshly squeezed lemon juice
2 Tbsp. olive oil
2 tsp. finely chopped dill
2 tsp. dijon mustard ✓
½ tsp. salt

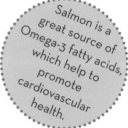

Salmon is a great source of Omega-3 fatty acids, which help to promote cardiovascular health.

Preheat grill to medium temperature.

BROWN RICE:
Follow instructions on package.

SALMON:
Rinse and pat dry salmon fillets. Place fillets skin side down. Grill approximately 10-15 minutes, or until fish flakes easily with a fork. Remove from heat.

SNOW PEAS:
Rinse snow peas. Steam or boil for 3-4 minutes or until tender.

LEMON DILL SAUCE:
In a small bowl, combine all lemon dill sauce ingredients. Whisk with a fork.

Drizzle lemon dill sauce over salmon fillets, snow peas and rice. Enjoy!

✓ *Please make sure this product is gluten-free.*
For specific brand name gluten-free products please see page 167.

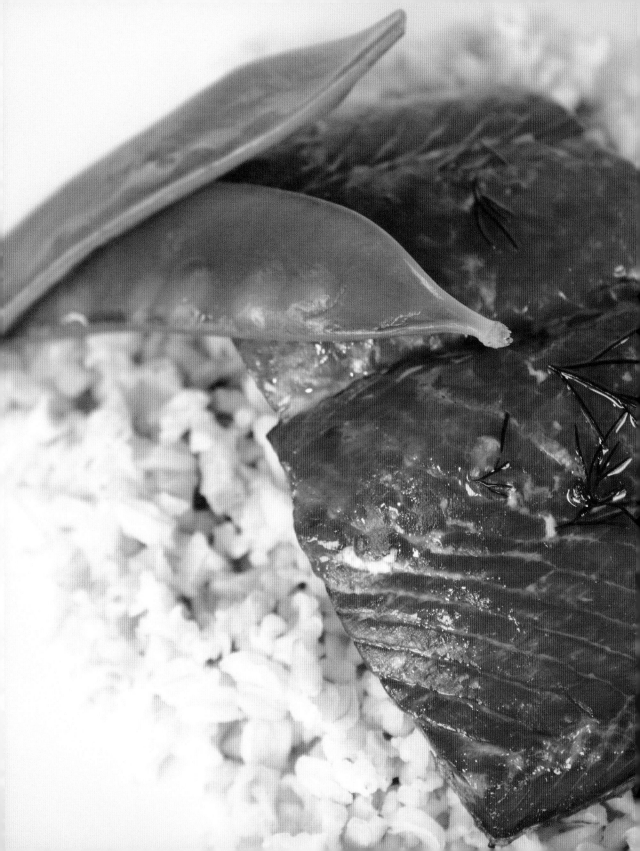

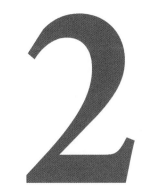

TODAY'S MENU: Day 2

BREAKFAST
....
Banana Pineapple Smoothie

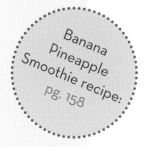

Banana Pineapple Smoothie recipe: pg. 158

SNACK
(optional)
....
Roasted & Salted Nuts ✔

LUNCH
....
Turkey Sandwich ✔ *with Potato Chips* ✔

SNACK
(optional)
....
Applesauce

DINNER
....
Stir-Fried Chicken & Vegetables in Gluten-Free Teriyaki Sauce ✔ *with Brown Rice*

SNACK
(optional)
....
Fresh Pineapple Slices

✔ *Please make sure this product is gluten-free.*
For specific brand name gluten-free products please see page 167.

LEMON DILL SAUCE

TERIYAKI SAUCE

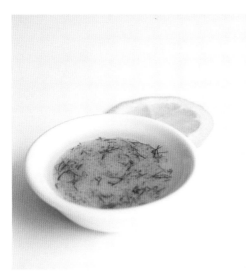

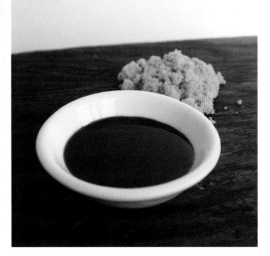

2 Tbsp. freshly squeezed lemon juice
2 Tbsp. olive oil
2 tsp. finely chopped dill
2 tsp. dijon mustard☑
½ tsp. salt

In a small bowl, combine all
ingredients. Whisk with a fork.
Serves 2.

2 Tbsp. olive oil
¼ cup gluten-free soy sauce☑
½ cup brown sugar

In a small sauté pan, heat olive oil
over medium/high temperature. Add
gluten-free soy sauce and brown
sugar. Bring to a boil. Reduce heat
and allow to simmer for 1 minute or
until sauce thickens.
Serves 2.

MASHED POTATOES   OVEN BAKED FRIES

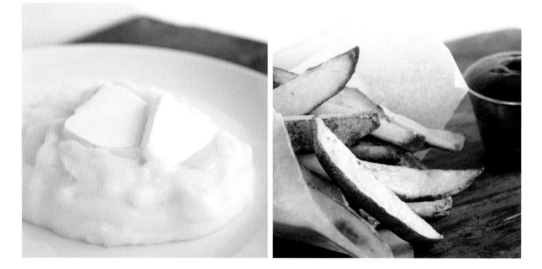

2 large russet potatoes
½ cup 2% milk
2 Tbsp. butter✓
½ tsp. onion salt

Peel and cube potatoes. In a medium
sauce pan, boil potatoes in water
for 15-20 minutes, or until soft. Drain
and place in a mixing bowl. Add milk,
butter, and onion salt. Blend or mash
to desired consistency.
Serves 2.

2 large russet potatoes
3 Tbsp. olive oil
salt to taste
freshly ground black pepper to taste

Preheat oven to 425 degrees.
Rinse and pat dry potatoes. Cut
potatoes into long thin strips. Place in
a large ziplock bag. Add olive oil. Shake
until potatoes are evenly coated with
olive oil. Spread potatoes out evenly
on a baking sheet. Bake 30-35 minutes
or until golden brown, flipping once.
Season with salt and pepper.
Serves 2.

SWEET POTATO FRIES

TACO SEASONING MIX

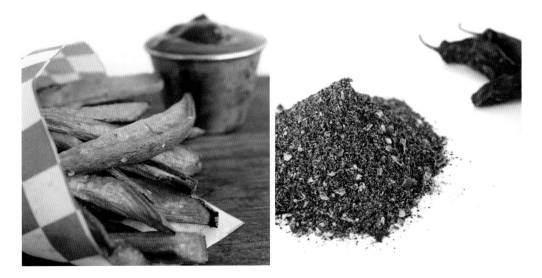

2 large sweet potatoes
3 Tbsp. olive oil
salt to taste
freshly ground black pepper to taste

Preheat oven to 425 degrees.
Rinse and pat dry sweet potatoes. Cut
into long thin strips. Place in a large
ziplock bag. Add olive oil. Shake until
potatoes are evenly coated with olive
oil. Spread potatoes out evenly on
a baking sheet. Bake 20-25 minutes
or until golden brown, flipping once.
Season with salt and pepper.
Serves 2.

1 ½ tsp. chili powder
⅛ tsp. garlic powder
⅛ tsp. onion powder
⅛ tsp. crushed red pepper
⅛ tsp. dried oregano
¼ tsp. paprika
¼ tsp. ground cumin
½ tsp. salt
½ tsp. minced onion flakes
1 tsp. rice flour

In a small bowl, mix all ingredients
together. Equivalent to ½ store
bought taco seasoning packet.
Serves 2.

ARTICHOKE

STEP 1   STEP 2

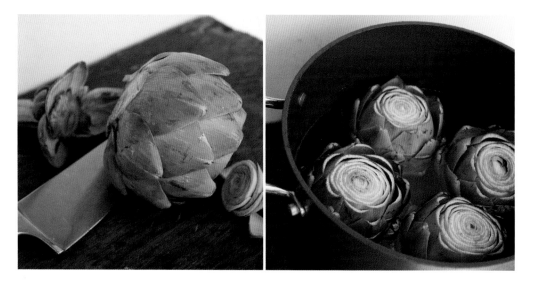

Cut off artichoke stem and ¾ inch   Boil or steam for 40-45 minutes.
off the artichoke tip.

STEP 3

STEP 4

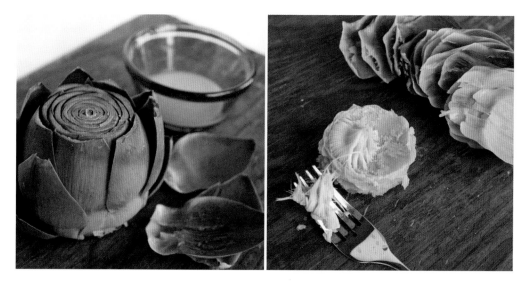

To eat the artichoke, individually pull off each leaf, starting with the outer leaves. Dip the white soft end into melted butter. Run teeth through inner soft edible portion of the leaf. Continue for all remaining leaves until you reach the artichoke heart.

Once all leaves are removed. Scrape out the inedible, fuzzy portion covering the artichoke heart.
The remaining bottom part is the artichoke heart. Cut into pieces and dip into melted butter.

MINI GLUTEN-FREE GROCERY SHOPPING GUIDE

MINI GLUTEN-FREE GROCERY SHOPPING GUIDE

....

For our full list of gluten-free grocery products, you may be interested in purchasing *Cecelia's Marketplace Gluten-Free Grocery Shopping Guide*. Please visit: www.CeceliasMarketplace.com

A

APPLES: *All **fresh** fruits & vegetables are gluten-free*

APPLESAUCE:
    Lucky Leaf - Cinnamon, Natural, Regular
    Mott's - Chunky, Cinnamon, Homestyle, Natural No Sugar Added, Original
    Musselman's - Chunky, Cinnamon, Homestyle, Organic, Regular, Unsweetened

ARTICHOKES: *All **fresh** fruits & vegetables are gluten-free*

ASPARAGUS: *All **fresh** fruits & vegetables are gluten-free*

AVOCADO: *All **fresh** fruits & vegetables are gluten-free*

B

BACON:
    Applegate Farms - Organic (Sunday, Turkey)
    Eckrich - Fully Cooked Ready To Crisp Bacon
    Jennie-O Turkey Store - Bacon (Extra Lean Turkey, Turkey)
    Jones Dairy Farm - Canadian, Sliced (Regular, Thick)
    Oscar Mayer - America's Favorite, Fully Cooked (Bacon, Thick Cut), Lower Sodium

BAKED BEANS:
    Bush's Best - Baked Beans (Bold & Spicy, Country Style, Homestyle, Original, Vegetarian)

BANANAS: *All **fresh** fruits & vegetables are gluten-free*

(B)

BARS:
    Bumble Bar - Awesome Apricot, Cherry Chocolate, Original Flavor
    Clif Nectar - Organic (Cherry Pomegranate, Cranberry Apricot Almond, Lemon Vanilla Cashew)
    Eat Natural - Cranberries Macadamias & Dark Chocolate, Macadamias Brazils & Apricots, Peanuts Almonds & Hazelnuts
    Enjoy Life - Caramel Apple, Cocoa Loco, Sunbutter Crunch, Very Berry
    Larabar - Apple Pie, Cherry Pie, Chocolate Chip Cookie Dough, Key Lime Pie, Lemon Bar, Pecan Pie, Peanut Butter Cookie

BBQ SAUCE:
    Jack Daniel's - Hickory Brown Sugar, Masterblend, Original No.7 Recipe, Smooth Original, Spicy Original
    Organicville - Organic BBQ Sauce (Original, Tangy)
    Sweet Baby Ray's - Hickory & Brown Sugar, Honey, Original, Sweet 'N Spicy

BEER:
    Anheuser-Busch - Redbridge Beer
    Bard's - American Lager
    Lakefront Brewery - New Grist Beer
    New Planet - 3R Raspberry Ale, Tread Lightly Ale

BELL PEPPERS: *All **fresh** fruits & vegetables are gluten-free*

BLUEBERRIES: *All **fresh** fruits & vegetables are gluten-free*

BOURBON: *All **distilled** alcohol is gluten-free*

BREAD:
  MIXES:
    1-2-3 Gluten Free - Aaron's Favorite Rolls, Meredith's Marvelous Muffin/Quickbread Mix
    Breads From Anna - All Purpose, Classic Herb, Gluten Free, Original
    Chebe - Bread Mix (All Purpose, Original), Frozen Dough (Rolls, Sandwich Buns)
    Gluten Free Pantry - Favorite Sandwich Bread Mix, French Bread & Pizza Mix
    Pamela's Products - Gluten-Free Bread Mix
  SLICED: *(Usually found in the frozen foods section of your grocery store)*
    Against The Grain Gourmet - Original Baguette, Original Rolls
    Ener-G - Sliced Breads (Light (Brown Rice, Tapioca, White Rice, White Rice Flax), White (Regular, Rice Flax), Yeast Free (Brown Rice, White Rice))
    Food For Life - Brown Rice, White Rice
    Kinnikinnick - Brown Sandwich, Sunflower Flax Rice, Tapioca Rice Original, White Sandwich, Yeast Free Tapioca

BREAD: (CONT.)

Rudi's Gluten-Free Bakery - Multigrain, Original
Schar - Baguette, Bread (Classic White, Multigrain), Rolls (Classic White, Sub Sandwich Rolls)
Udi's Gluten Free Foods - Gluten Free (White Sandwich, Whole Grain Loaf)

BROCCOLI: *All **fresh** fruits and vegetables are gluten-free*

BROWN RICE...SEE RICE

BROWN SUGAR...SEE SUGAR

BUTTER:

Earth Balance - Natural Buttery Spread (Olive Oil, Original, Soy Free, Soy Garden)
I Can't Believe It's Not Butter - Light, Original
Land-O-Lakes - Salted Butter, Unsalted Butter

C

CANDY/CANDY BARS:

Hershey's - Heath Bar, Mr. Goodbar, PayDay, Reese's Peanut Butter Cups (Original)
Lifesavers - All Varieties
M & M's - Almond, Dark Chocolate, Milk Chocolate, Peanut
Nestle - Baby Ruth, Oh Henry
Skittles - All Varieties
Snickers - Dark, Original
Starburst - All Varieties

CARAMEL DIP:

Litehouse - Low Fat Caramel, Original Caramel
Marzetti - Caramel Apple (Fat Free, Light, Old Fashioned)

CEREAL:

Chex - Chocolate, Cinnamon, Corn, Honey Nut, Rice
Cocoa Pebbles
EnviroKidz - Organic (Amazon Frosted Flakes, Gorilla Munch, Koala Crisp, Peanut Butter Panda Puffs)
Fruity Pebbles
Rice Krispies (Box must say "Gluten-Free")

CHAMPAGNE: *All champagne/sparkling wine **made in the US** is gluten-free*

CHEESE:

Athenos - Traditional Feta
Belgioioso - Parmesan

Boar's Head - All Varieties

Kraft -
Natural Shredded (Colby & Monterey Jack (2% Milk, Finely Shredded, Regular), Mexican Four Cheese, Monterey Jack)
Shredded Parmesan *(Plastic Container)*
Shredded Parmesan & Romano *(Plastic Container)*
Singles 2% Milk (American, Pepperjack, Sharp Cheddar, Swiss)
Singles Deli Deluxe (American, Sharp Cheddar)
Singles Fat Free (American, Sharp Cheddar, Swiss)
Singles Regular (American, Sharp Cheddar)

Organic Valley - Cheddar (Mild, Sharp), Colby, Feta, Mexican Blend Shredded, Monterey Jack (Reduced Fat, Regular), Mozzarella, Muenster, Pepper Jack

Sara Lee - Slices (American, Baby Swiss, Hot Pepper Monterey Jack, Longhorn Colby, Longhorn Colby Jack, Mild Cheddar, Mozzarella, Muenster, Smoked Provolone)

Sargento -
Artisan Blends Shredded (Parmesan, Parmesan Romano)
Classic Blends Shredded (4 Cheese Mexican, 6 Cheese Italian)
Classic Fancy Shredded (Colby Jack, Mild Cheddar, Monterey Jack, Mozzarella, Sharp Cheddar)
Deli Style (Baby Swiss, Chipotle Cheddar, Colby, Colby Jack)
Reduced Fat Deli Style (Colby Jack, Medium Cheddar, Pepper Jack)
Reduced Fat Shredded (4 Cheese Italian, 4 Cheese Mexican, Colby Jack, Mild Cheddar, Mozzarella, Sharp Cheddar)

CHICKEN: All *fresh* chicken is gluten-free (non-marinated, unseasoned)

CHIPS:
Baked Lay's - Original, Sour Cream & Onion
Baked Ruffles - Cheddar & Sour Cream, Original
Doritos - Cool Ranch
Eat Smart - Garden Veggie Crisps
Fritos - Original Corn Chips
Kettle Brand - Potato Chips (Backyard Barbeque, Sea Salt & Vinegar, Sour Cream Onion & Chive, Unsalted)
Lay's - Potato Chips (Classic, Lightly Salted, Salt & Vinegar, Sour Cream & Onion)
Lay's Stax - Potato Crisps (Mesquite Barbecue, Original, Salt & Vinegar, Sour Cream & Onion)
Lundberg - Rice Chips (Nacho Cheese, Pico De Gallo, Sea Salt)
Riceworks - Gourmet Brown Rice Crisps (Salsa Fresca, Sea Salt, Tangy BBQ)
Ruffles - Original (Light, Reduced Fat, Regular)
Wise - Potato Chips (All Natural, Lightly Salted, Salt & Vinegar, Unsalted)

CIDER:
- **Lucky Leaf** - Apple Cider, Sparkling Apple Cider
- **Magners** - Cider *(Alcoholic)*
- **Musselman's** - Cider, Fresh Pressed, Sparkling Cider
- **Woodchuck Hard Cider** - Hard Cider (All Varieties) *(Alcoholic)*
- **Wyder's** - Hard Cider (All Varieties) *(Alcoholic)*

CILANTRO: *All **fresh & pure** herbs are gluten-free*

CLUB SODA:
- **Canada Dry** - All Varieties
- **Schweppes** - All Varieties

COD: *All **fresh** fish is gluten-free (non-marinated, unseasoned)*

COFFEE:
- **Folger's** - All Instant & Roasts
- **Maxwell House** -
  - Coffee Bags (Decaf, Master Blend, Regular)
  - Filter Packs & Singles (Decaf, Original)
  - French Vanilla (Regular, Sugar Free, Sugar Free & Decaffeinated)
  - Ground (All Varieties)
- **Nescafe** - Classic Instant, Singles (All Varieties), Taster's Choice (All Varieties)

COLESLAW: *All **fresh** fruits and vegetables are gluten-free*

COLESLAW DRESSING:
- **Litehouse** - Regular Coleslaw Dressing
- **Walden Farms** - Sugar Free No Carb Coleslaw Dressing

CORN CHIPS...SEE CHIPS

CORN ON THE COB: *All **fresh** fruits and vegetables are gluten-free*

CORN TORTILLAS...SEE TORTILLAS

CRACKERS:
- **Blue Diamond** - Nut Thins (Cheddar Cheese, Country Ranch, Hint Of Sea Salt, Smokehouse)
- **Crunchmaster** - Multi Grain (Five Seed, Original), Multi Seed (Original, Toasted Onion)
- **Edward & Sons** - Brown Rice Snaps (Black Sesame, Cheddar, Onion Garlic, Toasted Onion, Unsalted Plain, Unsalted Sesame, Vegetable)
- **Glutino** - Gluten Free Crackers (Multigrain, Original, Table, Vegetable)
- **Mary's Gone Crackers** - Black Pepper, Caraway, Herb, Onion, Original

Looking for more gluten-free products? Cecelia's Marketplace Gluten-Free Grocery Shopping Guide contains thousands of GF products.

CREAM OF RICE:
  Nabisco - Cream of Rice

CUCUMBERS: *All **fresh** fruits & vegetables are gluten-free*

D

DELI MEAT:
  Applegate Farms - All Varieties
  Boar's Head - All Varieties
  Carl Buddig - Original (Beef, Brown Sugar Ham, Ham, Honey Ham, Honey Roasted Turkey, Mesquite Turkey, Oven Roasted Turkey, Turkey)
  Dietz & Watson - Cooked Ham, Genoa Salami, Smoked Maple Ham
  Eckrich - Lunch Meat (Hard Salami, Virginia Brand Thin Sliced Ham)
  Hillshire Farms -
    Deli Select (Baked Ham, Honey Ham, Honey Roasted Turkey Breast, Oven Roasted Turkey Breast, Roast Beef, Smoked Turkey Breast)
    Deli Select Ultra Thin (Hard Salami, Honey Ham, Honey Roasted Turkey Breast, Mesquite Smoked Turkey, Oven Roasted Turkey Breast, Smoked Ham)
  Hormel - Natural Choice (Cooked Deli Ham, Deli Roast Beef, Hard Salami, Honey Deli (Ham, Turkey), Oven Roasted Deli Turkey, Smoked Deli (Ham, Turkey))
  Oscar Mayer - Shaved Deli Fresh Meats (French Dip Roast Beef, Honey Smoked Turkey Breast, Oven Roasted Turkey Breast, Slow Roasted Roast Beef, Smoked Ham, Smoked Turkey Breast)

DIJON MUSTARD...SEE MUSTARD

DILL: *All **fresh & pure** herbs are gluten-free*

DRINKS:
  Campbell's - Tomato Juice (Healthy Request, Low Sodium, Organic, Original)
  Capri Sun - All Varieties
  Country Time - Lemonade
  Dole - All Fruit Juice
  Hawaiian Punch - All Varieties
  Juicy Juice - Fruit Juice (All Flavors), Sparkling Fruit Juice (All Flavors)
  Minute Maid - Lemonade (Light, Original)
  Mott's - All Varieties
  Ocean Spray - All Varieties
  Simply - Apple, Lemonade (Original, w/Raspberry), Orange
  Sunny D - All Varieties
  Tropicana - All 100% Juices
  V8 - 100% Vegetable Juice

E

EGGS: *All **fresh** eggs are gluten-free*

F

FRENCH FRIES:
> **Ore-Ida** - Cottage Fries, Extra Crispy Golden Crinkles, Golden (Crinkles, Fries), Shoestrings, Steak Fries, Sweet Potato Fries, Waffle Fries
> **Woodstock Farms** - Organic Crinkle Cut Oven Fries

FRUIT CUP:
> **Del Monte** - Canned/Jarred Fruit (All Varieties), Fruit Snack Cups (Metal, Plastic)

G

GARLIC: *All **fresh** garlic is gluten-free*

GELATIN:
> **Jell-O** -
> Regular (Cherry, Grape, Lemon, Raspberry, Strawberry, Watermelon)
> Sugar Free Low Calorie (Cherry, Mixed Fruit, Orange, Raspberry, Strawberry)
> **Kool-Aid** - Gels (All Varieties)
> **Royal** - All Varieties

GIN: *All **distilled** alcohol is gluten-free*

GREEN BEANS: *All **fresh** fruits and vegetables are gluten-free*

GROUND BEEF: *All **fresh** ground beef is gluten-free (non-marinated, unseasoned)*

GROUND TURKEY: *All **fresh** ground turkey is gluten-free (non-marinated, unseasoned)*

H

HAM:
> **Applegate Farms** - Natural (Black Forest, Honey), Organic Uncured Ham
> **Armour** - 1877 (Canadian Maple, Honey Cured, Virginia Baked)
> **Boar's Head** - All Varieties
> **Carl Buddig** - Deli Cuts (Baked Honey Ham, Brown Sugar Baked Ham, Smoked Ham), Original (Brown Sugar Ham, Honey Ham, Regular)
> **Dietz & Watson** - Breakfast Ham Fillets w/Water Added
> **Hillshire Farms** - Deli Select (Brown Sugar Baked Ham, Smoked Ham), Whole/Half (All Flavors)

Hormel - Black Label (Canned, Chopped), Ham Patties, Natural Choice (Cooked Deli, Honey, Smoked Deli)
SPAM - Classic, Hickory Smoke Flavored, Less Sodium, Lite

HAMBURGER BUNS: *(Usually found in the frozen foods section of your grocery store)*
Ener-G - Hamburger Buns (Tapioca, White Rice)
Rudi's Gluten-Free Bakery - Multigrain Hamburger Buns
Udi's Gluten Free Foods - Hamburger Buns (Classic, Whole Grain)

HASHBROWNS:
Ore-Ida - Hash Browns (Country Style, Golden Patties, Southern Style)
Woodstock Farms - Organic Frozen Shredded Hash Browns

I

ICE CREAM:
Breyer's - All Natural (Chocolate, Chocolate Chip, Mint Chocolate Chip, Strawberry, Vanilla)
Dreyer's - Fruit Bars (Grape, Pineapple, Strawberry, Tangerine)
Edy's - Fruit Bars (Grape, Pineapple, Strawberry, Tangerine)
Haagen-Dazs - Ice Cream (Chocolate, Mango, Mint Chip, Strawberry, Vanilla)
It's Soy Delicious - Chocolate Peanut Butter, Mango Raspberry, Raspberry, Vanilla
Purely Decadent - Dairy Free Ice Cream (Chocolate Obsession, Coconut Craze, Purely Vanilla, So Very Strawberry)
Soy Dream - French Vanilla, Mocha Fudge, Vanilla

J

JAMS/JELLIES:
Smuckers - All Jams & Jellies
Welch's - All Jams, Jellies & Preserves

JELLO...SEE GELATIN

JUICE...SEE DRINKS

K

KETCHUP:
Heinz - No Salt Added, Reduced Sugar, Regular
Organicville - Organic

L

LAMB CHOPS: *All **fresh** lamb is gluten-free (non-marinated, unseasoned)*

LEMONS: *All **fresh** fruits and vegetables are gluten-free*

LETTUCE: *All **fresh** lettuce is gluten-free*

LIMES: *All **fresh** fruits & vegetables are gluten-free*

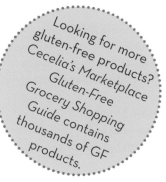

Looking for more gluten-free products? Cecelia's Marketplace Gluten-Free Grocery Shopping Guide contains thousands of GF products.

M

MANGO: *All **fresh** fruits and vegetables are gluten-free*

MARINARA SAUCE:
>   **Bertolli** - Marinara w/Burgundy Wine, Tomato & Basil
>   **Classico** - Cabernet Marinara w/Herbs, Roasted Garlic, Tomato & Basil, Traditional Sweet Basil
>   **Emeril's** - Home Style Marinara, Roasted (Gaahlic, Red Pepper), Tomato & Basil
>   **Newman's Own** - Cabernet Marinara, Marinara (Regular, w/Mushroom), Organic (Marinara, Tomato Basil), Sweet Onion & Roasted Garlic
>   **Prego** - Chunky Garden (Tomato Onion & Garlic), Fresh Mushroom, Heart Smart (Mushroom, Traditional), Marinara, Tomato Basil & Garlic, Traditional
>   **Ragu** -
>   Chunky (Garden Combination, Super Chunky Mushroom, Tomato Garlic & Onion)
>   Light (No Sugar Added Tomato & Basil, Tomato & Basil)
>   Old World Style (Marinara, Traditional)
>   Organic (Garden Veggie, Traditional)

MAYONNAISE:
>   **Best Foods** - Canola, Light, Low Fat, Real, w/Lime Juice
>   **Hellmann's** - Canola, Light, Olive Oil Mayo Dressing, Real, Reduced Fat
>   **Kraft** - Real Mayo
>   **Miracle Whip** - Free, Light, Regular

MILK: *All **fresh** milk is gluten-free (unflavored)*

MILK ALTERNATIVES:
>   **A Taste of Thai** - Coconut Milk (Lite, Regular)
>   **Blue Diamond** - Refrigerated Almond Breeze (Chocolate, Original, Unsweetened Vanilla, Vanilla), Shelf Stable Almond Breeze (Chocolate, Original, Vanilla), Shelf Stable Almond Breeze Unsweetened (Chocolate, Original, Vanilla)
>   **Pacific Natural Foods** - Almond Milk (Chocolate, Low Fat Original, Low Fat Vanilla, Unsweetened Original, Unsweetened Vanilla), Rice Milk (Low Fat Plain, Low Fat Vanilla), Soy Milk (All Varieties)

Rice Dream - Refrigerated & Shelf Stable Rice Beverages (All Varieties)
Silk Soymilk - All Varieties
Soy Dream - Shelf Stable Enriched (Chocolate, Original, Vanilla)
Thai Kitchen - Coconut Milk (Lite, Regular)

MUSHROOMS: *All **fresh** fruits and vegetables are gluten-free*

MUSTARD:
Emeril's - Dijon, Smooth Honey, Yellow
French's - Classic Yellow, Honey, Honey Dijon, Spicy Brown
Grey Poupon - Deli, Dijon, Hearty Spicy Brown, Savory Honey

N
NUTS:
Blue Diamond - 100 Calorie Almond Packs (Lightly Salted, Sea Salt, Whole Natural)
Emerald - On The Go Canisters (Cashews Halves & Pieces, Dry Roasted Almonds,
    Dry Roasted Peanuts)
Planters -
    Almonds (Dry Roasted)
    Mixed (Cashew Lovers, Honey Roasted, Lightly Salted, Regular)
    Nut-rition (Almonds, Antioxidant, Digestive Health, Heart Healthy)
    Peanuts (Honey Roasted, Unsalted)

O
OIL:
Bertolli - Olive Oil (Classico, Extra Light, Extra Virgin)
Crisco - Canola w/Omega 3DHA, Frying Blend, Natural Blend, Olive
    (100% Extra Virgin, Light Tasting, Pure), Pure (Canola, Corn, Peanut, Vegetable)
Filippo Berio - Extra Virgin Olive
Mazola - Canola Oil, Corn Oil, Corn Oil Plus, Olive Oil (Extra Virgin, Pure),
    Vegetable Plus

OLIVE OIL...SEE OIL

OLIVES:
B&G - Black, Greek
Mezzetta - Calamata (Greek, Pitted, Sliced), Salad, Spanish (Colossal Queen
    w/Minced Pimento, Manzanilla w/Minced Pimento, Queen Martini In Dry Vermouth)
Tassos - Black Olives In Extra Virgin Olive Oil & Red Wine, Kalamata In Tassos Extra
    Virgin Olive Oil & Red Wine Vinegar

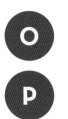

ONION SALT:
    Durkee
    McCormick
    Spice Islands
    Tones

ONIONS: *All **fresh** fruits and vegetables are gluten-free*

P

PAPAYA: *All **fresh** fruits and vegetables are gluten-free*

PARMESAN CHEESE...SEE CHEESE

PARSLEY: *All **fresh & pure** herbs are gluten-free*

PASTA:
    Ancient Harvest Quinoa - Quinoa Pasta (Shells, Spaghetti, Veggie Curls)
    DeBoles - Corn Pasta Spaghetti, Gluten Free Rice Pasta (Angel Hair, Spaghetti, Spirals)
    Schar - Penne, Spaghetti
    Tinkyada - Brown Rice (Penne, Shells, Spaghetti, Spirals), Organic Brown Rice (Penne, Spaghetti, Spirals)

PASTA SAUCE...SEE MARINARA SAUCE

PEPPER:
    Durkee - All Pepper Black/White
    McCormick - All Pepper Black/White
    Spice Islands - All Pepper Black/White
    Tones - All Pepper Black/White

PICKLES:
    Mt. Olive -
        Dills (Jumbo, Large, Original, Thin)
        Hamburger Dill Chips
        Kosher (Baby Dills, Dill Chips, Hamburger Dill Chips, Petite Dills, Zesty Garlic Dills)
        Sweet (Gerkins, Midgets, Pickles)
    Vlasic - All Varieties

PINEAPPLE: *All **fresh** fruits and vegetables are gluten-free*

POPCORN:
    Jolly Time - Microwave (Blast O Butter (Light, Regular), Healthy Pop (Butter Flavor, Kettle Corn, Regular))

Newman's Own - Microwave (Butter, Light Butter, Natural)
Newman's Own Organics - Microwave Pop's Corn (Butter Flavored, Light Butter Flavored)
Pop Secret - Microwave (Butter, Extra Butter, Kettle Corn, Light Butter, Movie Theater Butter)

POPSICLES:
Fla-Vor-Ice - Freezer Bars (Light, Regular, Sport, Tropical)
Icee - Freezer Bars
Pop Ice - Freezer Pops

PORK CHOPS: All *fresh* pork is gluten-free (non-marinated, unseasoned)

POTATO FLOUR:
Bob's Red Mill
Ener-G - Pure Potato Flour

POTATOES: All *fresh* fruits and vegetables are gluten-free

PUDDING:
Jell-O -
Regular Cook N' Serve (Banana Cream, Butterscotch, Chocolate, Lemon, Vanilla)
Regular Instant Pudding & Pie Filling (Banana Cream, Butterscotch, Chocolate, Lemon, Vanilla)
Kozy Shack - All Varieties (Flans, Gels, Puddings)

Q
QUINOA:
Ancient Harvest Quinoa - Inca Red Quinoa, Quinoa Flakes, Traditional Quinoa Grain
Arrowhead Mills - Quinoa
Eden Organic - Whole Grain Quinoa

R
RANCH DIP:
Lay's - Smooth Ranch Dip
Marzetti - Ranch (Fat Free, Light, Organic, Regular)

RED ONION: All *fresh* fruits and vegetables are gluten-free

RED PEPPER FLAKES:
Durkee - Crushed Red Pepper
McCormick - Crushed Red Pepper (Organic, Regular)

RED PEPPER FLAKES: (CONT.)

Spice Islands - Crushed Red Pepper
Tones - Crushed Red Pepper

RICE:

Fantastic World Foods - Arborio, Basmati, Jasmine
Lundberg - All Varieties
Minute Rice - Brown Rice, Ready To Serve Rice (Brown & Wild, Spanish, White, Whole Grain Brown, Yellow), Steamers (Spanish, White, Whole Grain Brown), White Rice
Success - Boil In Bag Rice (Jasmine, White, Whole Grain Brown)
Uncle Ben's - Boil In Bag, Instant Rice, Ready Rice (Original Long Grain Rice 8.8 oz. & 14.8 oz., Whole Grain Brown Rice)

RICE CAKES:

Lundberg - Eco Farmed Brown Rice (Lightly Salted, Toasted Sesame), Organic Brown Rice (Lightly Salted, Salt Free)
Quaker - Butter Popcorn, Lightly Salted, Unsalted, White Cheddar

RICE CHIPS...SEE CHIPS

RICE FLOUR:

Bob's Red Mill - Organic (Brown Rice, White Rice), Sweet Rice, White Rice
Ener-G - Brown Rice, Sweet Rice, White Rice

RUM: *All **distilled** alcohol is gluten-free*

S

SALAD: *All **fresh** lettuce is gluten-free*

SALAD DRESSING:

Drew's - Buttermilk Ranch, Garlic Italian Vinaigrette, Romano Caesar
Ken's Steakhouse -
Light Options (Italian w/Romano & Red Pepper, Ranch, Raspberry Walnut)
Regular (Caesar, Greek, Italian & Marinade, Ranch, Zesty Italian)
Kraft - Classic Caesar, Greek Vinaigrette, Light Raspberry Vinaigrette, Ranch, Zesty Italian
Litehouse - Caesar, Ranch, Raspberry Walnut Vinaigrette, Zesty Vinaigrette Italian
Newman's Own - Caesar, Creamy Italian, Greek Vinaigrette, Ranch
Wish-Bone - Italian (Fat Free, Light, Regular), Ranch (Light, Regular), Raspberry Hazelnut Vinaigrette

SALAMI...SEE DELI MEAT

SALMON: *All **fresh** fish is gluten-free (non-marinated, unseasoned)*

S

SALSA:
Chi-Chi's - Original
Newman's Own - All Natural (Hot, Medium, Mild), Black Bean & Corn
Old El Paso - Thick N' Chunky (Hot, Medium, Mild)
Ortega - Black Bean & Corn, Garden Vegetable (Medium, Mild), Original (Medium, Mild), Thick & Chunky (Medium, Mild)
Pace - Chunky (Medium, Mild), Thick & Chunky (Extra Mild, Hot, Medium, Mild)
Tostitos - All Natural Chunky (Hot, Medium, Mild), Restaurant Style

SALT:
Morton - Coarse Kosher, Iodized Table, Plain Table, Salt Substitute, Sea Salt (Coarse, Fine)

SAUSAGE:
Jennie-O Turkey Store - Fresh Breakfast Sausage (Maple Links, Mild Links, Mild Patties)
Jimmy Dean - Heat 'N Serve Sausage Links (Hot, Maple, Original), Heat 'N Serve Sausage Patties
Johnsonville - Original Breakfast Sausage (Links, Patties), Vermont Maple Syrup Breakfast Sausage (Links, Patties)
Jones Dairy Farm -
All Natural Sausage (Hearty Pork Links, Light Pork & Rice Links, Little Links Pork, Maple Links)
Golden Brown All Natural Fully Cooked (Beef Sausage Links, Maple Sausage (Links, Patties), Mild Sausage (Links, Patties))

SELTZER:
Canada Dry - All Varieties
Schweppes - All Varieties

SHRIMP: *All **fresh** seafood is gluten-free (non-marinated, unseasoned)*

SNACK BARS...SEE BARS

SNOW PEAS: *All **fresh** fruits and vegetables are gluten-free*

SODA POP:
7up - All Varieties
A & W - Root Beer
Barq's Root Beer - Caffeine Free, Diet, Regular
Coca-Cola -
Cherry Coke (Diet, Regular, Zero)
Classic Coke (Caffeine Free, Regular, Zero)
Diet Coke (Caffeine Free, Plus, Regular, w/Lime, w/Splenda)
Vanilla Coke (Regular, Zero)

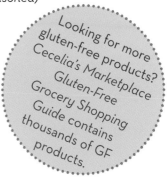

Looking for more gluten-free products? Cecelia's Marketplace Gluten-Free Grocery Shopping Guide contains thousands of GF products.

SODA POP: (CONT.)

S

Crush - Cherry, Grape, Orange, Strawberry
Dr. Pepper - All Varieties
Fanta - Grape, Orange
Hires - Root Beer
I.B.C. - Root Beer
Mountain Dew - Caffeine Free, Caffeine Free Diet, Diet, Regular
Mr. Pibb - Xtra, Zero
Mug - Cream Soda (Diet, Regular), Root Beer (Diet, Regular)
Pepsi - Caffeine Free Pepsi (Diet, Regular), Cherry Vanilla, Pepsi (Diet, Regular)
Sprite - Regular, Zero
Squirt - All Varieties
Sunkist - Diet Orange, Fruit Punch, Grape, Orange, Peach, Strawberry
Welch's - All Varieties

SORBET:

Haagen-Dazs - Sorbet (Mango, Orchard Peach, Raspberry, Strawberry, Zesty Lemon)
So Delicious - Coconut Water Sorbet (Hibiscus, Lemonade, Mango, Raspberry)

SOUP:

Dr. McDougall's - Ready To Serve Soups (Chunky Tomato, Roasted Pepper Tomato, Vegetable), Soup Cup (Light Sodium Split Pea)
Imagine -
   Organic Creamy (Sweet Pea, Tomato, Tomato Basil)
   Organic Creamy Light In Sodium (Garden Tomato & Basil)
Kettle Cuisine - Frozen Soup Bowls (Chicken w/Rice Noodles, New England Clam Chowder, Roasted Vegetable)
Pacific Natural Foods -
   Organic Creamy (Creamy Roasted Red Pepper & Tomato, Creamy Tomato)
   Organic Light Sodium (Creamy Tomato, Roasted Red Pepper & Tomato)
   Organic Savory Chicken & Wild Rice
   Organic Split Pea w/Ham & Swiss Cheese
Progresso - Traditional (Chicken Rice & Vegetables, New England Clam Chowder, Split Pea w/Ham), Vegetable Classics (Garden Vegetable)
Simply Asia - Spring Vegetable Rice Noodle Soup Bowl
Thai Kitchen - Garlic & Vegetable Instant Rice Noodle Soup
Wolfgang Puck - Tomato Basil Bisque

SOUR CREAM:

Breakstone - All Natural, Fat Free, Reduced Fat
Daisy Brand - Fat Free, Light, Regular
Horizon Organic - All Varieties
Organic Valley - Low Fat, Regular

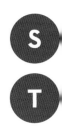

SOY SAUCE:
>   **Eden Organic** - Organic Tamari Soy Sauce *(Brewed In U.S.)*
>   **San-J** - Organic Tamari Wheat Free Soy Sauce (Reduced Sodium, Regular)

STEAK: *All **fresh** beef is gluten-free (non-marinated, unseasoned)*

STRAWBERRIES: *All **fresh** fruits & vegetables are gluten-free*

SUGAR:
>   **Domino** - Brown, Confectioners, Cubes, Granulated, Organic

SWEET POTATO FRIES...SEE FRENCH FRIES

SWEET POTATOES: *All **fresh** fruits and vegetables are gluten-free*

T

TACO SEASONING:
>   **Old El Paso** - Taco Seasoning Mix (Mild, Original)
>   **Ortega** - Hot & Spicy Mix, Taco 40% Less Sodium Mix, Taco Seasoning Mix

TACO SHELLS:
>   **Old El Paso** - Stand N' Stuff Yellow Corn Taco Shells, Taco Shells (White Corn, Yellow Corn)
>   **Ortega** - Hard Shells (White, Whole Grain, Yellow)

TEA:
>   **Arizona** - All Varieties
>   **Lipton** -
>   Bottled Iced Tea (Green w/Citrus, Iced Tea w/Lemon)
>   Green Tea Bags (100% Natural, 100% Natural Decaf)
>   Herbal Tea Bags (Lemon, Peppermint, Quietly Chamomile)
>   Iced Tea Mix (Lemon, Unsweetened, Wild Raspberry)
>   **Snapple** - All Varieties
>   **Tazo Tea** - All Varieties ***(Except Green Ginger & Tazo Honeybush)***

TEQUILA: *All **distilled** alcohol is gluten-free*

TILAPIA: *All **fresh** fish is gluten-free (non-marinated, unseasoned)*

TOMATOES: *All **fresh** fruits and vegetables are gluten-free*

TONIC WATER:
 Canada Dry - All Varieties
 Schweppes - All Varieties

TORTILLAS:
 French Meadow Bakery - Gluten Free Tortillas
 Mission - Corn Tortillas (Extra Thin, White, Yellow)

TUNA FISH:
 Bumble Bee -
  Chunk White Albacore (In Oil, In Water)
  Premium Albacore Tuna (In Water Pouch)
  Solid White Albacore (In Water)
 Chicken Of The Sea - All Products
 Crown Prince - Natural Albacore (Solid White, Solid White No Salt Added)
 StarKist -
  Canned
   Classics (All Varieties)
   Gourmet Choice (Albacore Tuna Fillet, Low Sodium, Solid Light Tuna
    Fillet In Olive Oil, Solid Light Tuna Fillet In Water)
  Pouch
   Albacore White (Low Sodium, Regular)
   Chunk Light (In Vegetable Oil, Low Sodium)

TURKEY...SEE DELI MEAT

U

V
VEGGIE CHIPS...SEE CHIPS

VODKA: *All **distilled** alcohol is gluten-free*

W
WATERMELON: *All **fresh** fruits & vegetables are gluten-free*

WHISKEY: *All **distilled** alcohol is gluten-free*

WHITE RICE...SEE RICE

WINE: *All wine **made in the US** is gluten-free*

X
Y

YOGURT:

Brown Cow Yogurt -
Low Fat (Blueberry, Peach, Plain 32, Strawberry, Vanilla 32)
Non Fat (Blueberry, Plain, Raspberry, Strawberry, Vanilla)
Whole Milk Yogurt (Blueberry, Plain, Raspberry, Strawberry, Vanilla)
Dannon - Plain (Low Fat, Natural, Non Fat)
Horizon Organic - All Varieties
Stonyfield Organic - All Frozen Yogurts, All Smoothies, All Soy Yogurts
WholeSoy & Co. - All Frozen Yogurts, All Smoothies, All Yogurts
Yoplait -
All Natural Plain Fat Free (16 oz., 32 oz.)
Light (Banana Cream Pie, Blackberry, Blueberry Patch, Key Lime Pie, Lemon Cream
Pie, Red Raspberry, Strawberries 'N Bananas, Strawberry, Very Cherry, Very Vanilla)
Light Fat Free (Creamy Strawberry, Creamy Vanilla)
Original (Banana Creme, Blackberry Harvest, Boysenberry, Cherry
Orchard, Harvest Peach, Key Lime Pie, Mango, Mixed Berry, Mountain
Blueberry, Pineapple, Red Raspberry, Strawberry)

Z

ZUCCHINI: *All **fresh** fruits and vegetables are gluten-free*

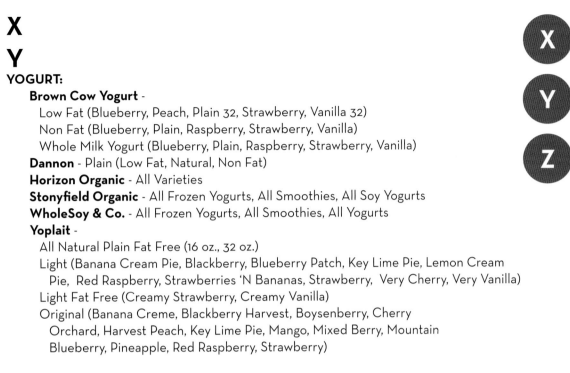

Looking for more gluten-free products? Cecelia's Marketplace Gluten-Free Grocery Shopping Guide contains thousands of GF products.

GLUTEN-FREE SPECIALTY PRODUCTS

1-2-3 Gluten-Free - www.123glutenfree.com
Against The Grain Gourmet - www.againstthegraingourmet.com
Ancient Harvest Quinoa - www.quinoa.net
Arrowhead Mills - www.arrowheadmills.com ★
Bob's Red Mill - www.bobsredmill.com ★
Breads From Anna - www.breadsfromanna.com
Chebe - www.chebe.com
Crunchmaster - www.crunchmaster.com
DeBoles - www.deboles.com ★
Ener-G - www.ener-g.com
Enjoy Life Foods - www.enjoylifefoods.com
Food For Life - www.foodforlife.com ★
French Meadow Bakery - www.frenchmeadow.com ★
Gluten-Free Pantry - www.glutenfree.com
Kettle Cuisine - www.kettlecuisine.com
Kinnikinnick - www.kinnikinnick.com
Mary's Gone Crackers - www.marysgonecrackers.com
Pamela's Products - www.pamelasproducts.com
Riceworks - www.riceworkssnacks.com
Rudi's Gluten-Free Bakery - www.rudisglutenfree.com ★
Schar - www.schar.com
San-J - www.san-j.com ★
Tinkyada - www.tinkyada.com
Udi's Gluten Free Foods - www.udisglutenfree.com ★

Be careful... Companies with the ★ symbol also sell products that contain gluten.

NOTES

_____
_____
_____
_____
_____
_____
_____
_____
_____
_____
_____
_____
_____
_____
_____
_____
_____
_____
_____
_____
_____
_____
_____
_____
_____
_____

Index

OTHER PRODUCTS BY CECELIA'S MARKETPLACE

Best Seller!

GLUTEN-FREE GROCERY SHOPPING GUIDE:
all products listed are gluten-free & wheat-free.

> **#1 Selling** Gluten-Free Grocery Shopping Guide Nationwide
> Time-saver for grocery shopping
> Small, compact and easy to carry (4.5" x 6.5")
> Lists thousands of gluten-free products
> Excellent for family members, friends, chefs, dietitians & others
> Symbols highlighting certified GF products & GF dedicated facilities

GLUTEN/CASEIN FREE GROCERY SHOPPING GUIDE:
all products listed are gluten-free, wheat-free, casein-free, milk-free & lactose free.

GLUTEN/CASEIN/SOY FREE GROCERY SHOPPING GUIDE:
all products listed are gluten-free, wheat-free, casein-free, milk-free, lactose-free & soy-free.

GLUTEN-FREE COOKBOOKS:
savory gluten-free international classic recipes

GLUTEN-FREE DINING OUT CARDS:
help educate your waiter & chef about what foods you can and cannot have. A must have for gluten-free dining out!

GLUTEN-FREE SAFETY LABELS:
help stop cross-contamination in your kitchen with large red stickers stating, "Gluten-Free! DO NOT CONTAMINATE"

Buy Online: **www.CeceliasMarketplace.com**